I0477313

HEALTH SERVICES DELIVERY AND ETHICAL IMPLICATIONS

HEALTH SERVICES DELIVERY AND ETHICAL IMPLICATIONS

ADAM A. MUSAH, PhD

HEALTH MANAGEMENT AND POLICY SPECIALIST

COPYRIGHT © 2016 BY ADAM A. MUSAH, PHD.

LIBRARY OF CONGRESS CONTROL NUMBER: 2015921384

ISBN:	HARDCOVER	978-1-5035-7714-5
	SOFTCOVER	978-1-5035-7713-8
	EBOOK	978-1-5035-7712-1

All rights reserved. No part of this book may be reproduced or transmitted in any form or by any means, electronic or mechanical, including photocopying, recording, or by any information storage and retrieval system, without permission in writing from the copyright owner.

Any people depicted in stock imagery provided by Thinkstock are models, and such images are being used for illustrative purposes only.
Certain stock imagery © Thinkstock.

Print information available on the last page.

Rev. date: 01/12/2016

To order additional copies of this book, contact:
Xlibris
1-888-795-4274
www.Xlibris.com
Orders@Xlibris.com
716915

CONTENTS

ABSTRACT

BREADTH

The objective of this module is to identify explore, and articulate the principles and assumptions behind contemporary issues and the ethical delivery of health services. The breadth component focuses on health services delivery and ethical implications in health care provision. Ethical topics addressed include: Ethics in Health Services Management, Theory of Justice, and Introduction to Ethical Theory. These publications explained the concept surrounding ethical dilemma in health care. Furthermore, I reviewed the following literature for further clarity on the subject matter: The American Counseling Association's ethical approach the code of ethics of the American Rheumatology which shed light on designing and supporting the college's mission and the code of ethics and professional responsibilities for healthcare ethics consultants.

ABSTRACT

DEPTH

The Depth section focuses on health services delivery and ethical decision-making. I reviewed 14 bibliographies on current health research findings, and some of the issues that triggered probing were: Assessment of harm potential and factors influencing patients' participation in decision-making, reducing premature infants' length of stay and improving patients' mental health outcome, and parental involvement in treatment decisions regarding their critical ill children. Some of the findings laid strong foundation for further research while others provided recommendations for rectifying ethical dilemma in health services delivery.

ABSTRACT

APPLICATION

The application component focuses on ethical theories applied in health services delivery. I applied the concept explored in the breath components and the analysis of findings on current research in the depth component and provided guidelines and recommendations. Adhering to these recommendations and or guidelines will help alleviate several ethical problems in the health care industry. Additionally, this project entails the critical review of the following publication: National and international approaches to ethical guidelines implementations and periodic evaluations, general health education on doctor and patient responsibilities and informed consent general consideration.

CONTEMPORARY ISSUES AND ETHICAL DELIVERY OF HEALTH SERVICES

Introduction

With a significant development of the health care industry comes along the growing awareness of the relevant ethical issues or ethical consideration in decision making (Levine, 2008). Ethics is relevant to all aspects of health care delivery system in addition to biomedical research that involves human subjects in the prospect of discovering new ways of benefiting people's health. Consequently, central to the process of health administration is the management of conflicting values, and the rapid changes that occur in our societies and health services field have made the task more challenging to manage. Therefore, all medical professionals and health researchers are required to undergo formal training in the theories and principles of ethics in health care (Levine 2008).

To clearly understand ethical issues and the strategies for managing them, I reviewed the following theories and models: Ethics in Health Services Management by Darr (1997), a Theory of Justice by Rawls (1971), and Introduction to Ethical Theory by Rogerson (1991). Additionally, I reviewed the following contemporary classical works on theories and general articles on ethical knowledge for in depth knowledge on ethics in health care: Group Counseling – Ethics and Professional Issues by Forester-Miller and Rubenstein, Making Hard Choices – Clarifying Controversial ethical issues, and A Practitioner's Guide to Mental Health Ethics by Haas and Malouf (1989).

This knowledge area module is designed for assistance in developing competence in the application of ethical theories and principles to decision making related to the provision and delivery of preventive, diagnostic, curative, and restorative level of health services to selected population. In other words, knowledge derived from selected readings will be helpful in strategizing an ethical management tool for health care organizations.

HEALTH SERVICES DELIVERY AND ETHICAL IMPLICATIONS

The following theories and models were reviewed to clarify various concepts shaping the ethical dilemma in the delivery of health services in the United States of America and other parts of the world. The classical works of Rawls, Joseph Fletcher and Immanuel Kant were compared and contrasted to clarify whether additional steps are required by our health care providers to address ethical concerns effectively. Some of these concerns may be about the impact of religion and cultural values on informed consent. Further, the issues of morality in ethical principles of health institutions were scrutinized to see if they impact one another.

Ethical Theories

If the practitioners of bioethics do not rely solely on cultural norms and emotions, what are their sources of determining what is right or wrong? The most comprehensive source is a theory of ethics, a broad set of moral principles or perhaps just one overriding principle that is used in measuring human conduct. Divine law is one such source, of course, but even in the Western religious traditions of bioethics both the Jewish and Catholic religions have rich and comprehensive commentaries on ethical issues, and the Protestant religion has a less cohesive but still important tradition, the law of God is interpreted in terms of human moral principles (Rawls, 1971). Recently bioethicists have paid more attention to analyzing the teachings of other religious traditions, such as Islam, Buddhism, Confucianism, and other eastern religions. A theory of ethics must be acceptable to many groups, not just the follower of one religious tradition. Most writers outside the religious traditions and some within them have looked to one of three major traditions in ethics: teleological theories, deontological theories, and natural law theories (Rawls, 1971).

Teleological Theories

Teleological theories are based on the idea that the end or purpose (from the Greek *telos,* or end) of the action determines its rightness or wrongness. The most prominent teleological theory is utilitarianism. In its simplest formulation, an act is moral if it brings more good consequences than bad ones. Utilitarian theories are derived from the works of two English philosophers: Jeremy Bentham (1748-1832) and John Stuart Mill (1806-1873 and Rawls, 1971). Rejecting the absolutist religious morality of his time, Bentham proposed that "utility" the greatest good for the greatest number should guide the actions of human beings. Invoking the hedonistic philosophy of Epicurean Greeks, Bentham said that pleasure *(hedon* in Greek) is good and pain is bad. Therefore, actions are right if they promote more pleasure than pain and wrong if they promote more pain than pleasure. Mill found the highest utility in "happiness," rather than pleasure. Mill's philosophy is echoed in the Declaration of Independence's espousal of "life, liberty, and the pursuit of happiness." Other utilitarian have looked to a range of utilities, or goods including friendship, love, devotion, and the like that they believe ought to be weighed in the balance to the utilitarian calculus.

Utilitarianism has a pragmatic appeal. It is flexible, and it seems impartial. However, its critics point out that utilitarianism can be used to justify suppression of individual rights for the good of society "the ends justify the means" and that it is difficult to quantify and compare "utilities," however they are defined. Utilitarianism, in its many forms, has had a powerful influence on bioethical discussion, partly because it is the closest to the case-by-case risk/benefit ratio that physicians use in clinical decision-making. Joseph Fletcher, a Protestant theologian who was one of the pioneers in bioethics in the 1950s, developed utilitarian theories that he called *situation ethics.* He argued that a true Christian morality does not blindly follow moral rules but acts from love and sensitivity to the particular situation and the needs of those involved. He has enthusiastically supported most modern technologies on the grounds that they lead to good ends (Rawls, 1971). According to Rogerson (1991), writers in this volume who use utilitarian theories to arrive at their moral judgments include Lawrence O. Gostin, who defends giving public health agencies sweeping powers in a bioterrorist threat; and Jerod M. Loeb and his colleagues, who defend animal experimentation.

Deontological Theories

The second major type of ethical theory is deontological. It holds true that the rightness or wrongness of an act should be judged on whether or not it conforms to a moral principle or rule, not on whether it leads to good or bad consequences (Rogerson K. 1991). The primary exponent of a deontological theory was Immanuel Kant (1724-1804), a German philosopher Kant declared that there is an ultimate norm, or supreme duty, which he called the "Moral Law." He held that an act is moral only if it springs from a "good will," the only thing that is good without qualification.

We must do good things, said Kant, because we have a duty to do them, not because they result in good consequences or because they give us pleasure although that can happen as well. Kant constructed a formal "Categorical Imperative," the ultimate test of morality: Recognizing that this formulation was far from clear, Kant said the same thing in three other ways. He explained that a moral rule must be one that can serve as a guide for everyone's conduct; it must be one that permits people to treat each other as ends in themselves, not solely as means to another's ends; and it must be one that each person can impose on himself by his own will, not one that is solely imposed by the state, one's parents, or God. Kant's Categorical Imperative, in the simplest terms, says that all persons have equal moral worth and that no rule can be moral unless all people can apply it autonomously to all other human beings. Although on its own, Kant's Categorical Imperative is merely a formal statement with no moral content at all, he gave some examples of what he meant: "Do not commit suicide," and "Help others in distress." (Rogerson K. 1991).

Kantian ethics is criticized by many who note that Kant gives little guidance on what to do when ethical principles conflict, as they often do. Moreover, they say, his emphasis on autonomous decision-making and individual will neglects the social and communal context in which people live and make decisions. It leads to isolation and unreality. These criticisms notwithstanding, Kantian ethics has stimulated much current thinking in bioethics. In this volume, the idea that certain actions are in and of themselves right or wrong underlies, for example, Patrick Lee and Robert P. George's argument against abortion because it involves killing a human being; Tom Regan's opposition to animal research; and President's Council on Bioethics' opposition to federal funding of human stem cell research (Rogerson, 1991).

According to (Rosenbaun, 1982), two modern deontological theorists are philosophers John Rawls and Robert M. Veatch. In a Theory of Justice (1971), Rawls places the highest value on equitable distribution of society's resources. He believes that society has a fundamental obligation to correct the inequalities of historical circumstance and natural endowment of its least well off members. According to this theory, some action is good only if it benefits the least well off. It can also benefit others, but that is secondary. His social justice theory has influenced bioethical writings concerning the allocation of scarce resources. Veatch has applied Rawlsian principles to medical ethics. In his book, A Theory of Medical Ethics (1981), he offers a model of social contract among professionals, patients, and society that emphasizes mutual respect and responsibilities. This contract model will, he hopes, avoid the narrowness of professional codes of ethics and the generalities and ambiguities of more broadly based ethical theories (Rosenbaun, 1982).

Natural Law Theory

The third strain of ethical theory that is prominent in bioethics is natural law theory, first developed by St. Thomas Aquinas (1223-1274). According to this theory, actions are morally right if they accord with our nature as human beings. The attribute that is distinctively human is the ability to reason and to exercise intelligence. Thus, argues this theory, we can know the good, which is objective and can be learned through reason. References to natural law theory are prominent in the works of Catholic theologians and writers; they see natural law as ultimately derived from God but knowable through the efforts of human beings. The influence of natural law theory can be seen in the issues of human stem cell research and genetic enhancement, declared Thomas Aquinas (Rogerson, 1991).

Theory of Virtue

The theory of virtue, another ethical theory with deep roots in the Aristotelian tradition, has recently been revived in bioethics. This theory stresses not the morality of any particular actions or rules but the disposition of individuals to act morally, to be virtuous. In its modern version, its primary exponent is Alasdair MacIntyre, whose book After Virtue (1980) urges a return to the Aristotelian model. Gregory Pence has applied the theory of virtue directly to medicine in Ethical Options in Medicine (1980); he lists temperance in personal life, compassion for the suffering patient, professional competence, justice, honesty, courage, and practical judgment as the virtues that are most desirable in physicians. Although this theory has not yet been as fully developed in bioethics as the utilitarian or deontological theories, it is likely to have particular appeal for physicians, many of whom have resisted formal ethics education on the grounds that moral character is the critical factor and that one can best learn to be a moral physician by emulating one's mentors (Berg and Braddock, 2001).

Although various authors, in this volume and elsewhere, appeal in rather direct ways to either utilitarian or deontological theories, often the various types are combined. One may argue that both particular actions are immoral in and of itself and that it will have bad consequences, some commentators say even Kant used this argument. In fact, probably no single ethical theory is adequate to deal with ramifications of all the issues. In that case we can turn to a middle level of ethical discussion. Between the abstractions of ethical theories, Kant's Categorical Imperative, and the specifics of moral judgment is a range of ethical principles concepts that can be applied to particular cases (Berg and Braddock 2001).

Ethical Principles

In its four years of deliberation in the 1970s, the National Commission for the Protection of Human Subjects of Biomedical and Behavioral Research grappled with some of the most difficult issues facing researchers and society: When, if ever, is it ethical to do research on fetuses, on children, or on people in mental institutions? This commission, which was composed of people from various religious backgrounds, professions, and social strata, was finally able to agree on specific recommendations on these questions, but only after they had finished their work did the commissioners try to determine what ethical principles they had used in reaching a consensus. In their Belmont Report (1978), named after the conference center where they met to discuss this question, the commissioners outlined that respect for persons, beneficence, and justice are the three items that should govern the conduct of research with human beings. These three principles, they believed, are generally accepted in our cultural tradition and can serve as basic justifications for the many particular ethical prescriptions and evaluations of human action. Because of the principles' general acceptance and widespread applicability, they are at the basis of most bioethical discussion. Although philosophers argue about whether other principles preventing harm to others or loyalty, for example, ought to be accorded equal weight with these three or should be included under another umbrella, they agree that these principles are fundamental (Belmont Report 1978).

Respect for Persons

Respect for persons incorporates at least two basic ethical convictions, according to the Belmont Report. Individuals should be treated as autonomous agents, and persons with diminished autonomy are entitled to protection. The derivation from Kant is clear. Because human beings have the capacity for rational action and moral choice, they have a value independent of anything that they can do or provide to others. Therefore, they should be treated in a way that respects their independent choices and judgments. Respecting autonomy means giving weight to autonomous persons' considered opinions and choices, and refraining from interfering with their choices unless those choices are clearly detrimental to others. However, since the capacity for autonomy varies with age, mental disability, or other circumstances, those people whose autonomy is diminished must be protected - but only in ways that serve their interests and do not interfere with the level of autonomy that they do possess (Rawls, 1971).

Two important moral rules are derived from the ethical principle of respect for persons: informed consent and truth telling. Persons can exercise autonomy only when they have been fully informed about the range of options open to them, and the process of informed consent is generally considered to include the elements of information, comprehension, and voluntariness. Thus, a person can give informed consent to some medical procedure only if he or she has full information about the risks and benefits, understands them, and agrees voluntarily that is, without being coerced or pressured into agreement. Although the principle of informed consent has become an accepted moral rule and a legal one as well, it is difficult if not impossible-to achieve in a real-world setting. It can easily be turned into a legalistic parody or avoided altogether. But as a moral ideal, it serves to balance the unequal power of the physician and patient (Parker, 2007).

According to SophiaOmni (2012), truth telling is another important moral ideal derived from the principle of respect for persons.

On the Supposed Right to Lie From the Benevolent Motives: Kant stated that it is a duty to tell the truth. The notion of duty is inseparable from the notion of right. A duty is what in one being corresponds to the right of another. Where there are no rights there are no duties, but only towards him who has a right to the truth. But no man has a right to a truth that injures others. To tell the truth is a duty, but only towards him who has a right to the truth (p. 1).

Justice

The third ethical principle that is generally accepted is justice, which means "what is fair" or "what is deserved." The Belmont Report of 1979 indicated that an injustice occurs when some benefit to which a person is entitled is denied without good reason or when some burden is imposed unduly, and that the interpretation should be that equals should be treated equally. However, some distinctions - such as age, experience, competence, physical condition, and the like - can justify unequal treatment. Those who appeal to the principle of justice are most concerned about which distinctions can be made legitimately and which ones cannot.

According to Rawls (1971), one important derivative of the principle of justice is the recent emphasis on "rights" in bioethics. Given the successes in the 1960s and 1970s of civil rights movements in the courts and political arena, it is easy to understand the appeal of "rights talk." An emphasis on individual rights is part of the American tradition, in a way that emphasis on the "common good" is not. The language of rights has been prominent in the abortion debate, for instance, where the "right to life" has been pitted against the "right to privacy" or the "right to control one's body." The "right to health care" is a potent rallying cry, though it is one that is difficult to enforce legally. Although claims to rights may be effective in marshaling political support and in emphasizing moral ideals, those rights may not be the most effective way to solve ethical dilemmas. Our society, as philosopher Ruth Macklin has pointed out, has not yet agreed on a theory of justice in health care that will determine who has what kinds of rights and-the other side of the coin-who has the obligation to fulfill them (Rawls, 1971).

Analysis of Ethical Theories

These three fundamental ethical principles of respect for persons, beneficence, and justice will carry weight in ethical decision-making. But what happens when they conflict? On each side of the issues are writers who appeal, explicitly or implicitly, to one or more of these principles. For example, Jean Toal sees beneficence as paramount, and she would criminalize drug-using behavior by pregnant women in order to prevent harm to their fetuses. Lynn M. Paltrow finds such a policy unjust because it singles out certain risks and certain women for state intervention. Some of the issues are concerned with how to interpret a particular principle: Whether, for example, it is more or less beneficent to allow a physician to assist in suicide, or whether society's interest in obtaining transplantable organs for those who need them and allowing payment for them (Rosenbaum, 1982).

Will it ever be possible to resolve such fundamental divisions are those that are not merely matters of procedure or interpretation but of fundamental differences in principle? Lest the situation seem hopeless, consider that some consensus does seem to have been reached on questions that seemed equally tangled a few decades ago. The idea that government should play a role in regulating human subjects research was hotly debated, but it is now generally accepted - at least if the research is medical, not social or behavioral in nature, and is federally funded. Moreover, the appropriateness of using the criterion of brain death for determining the death of a person and the possibility of subsequent removal of their organs for transplantation has largely been accepted and written into state laws. The idea that a hopelessly ill patient has the legal and moral right to refuse treatment that will only postpone dying is also well established though it is often hard to exercise because hospitals and physicians continue to resist it. Finally, nearly everyone now agrees that health care is distributed unjustly in the United States - a radical idea only a few years ago. There is, of course, sharp disagreement about whose responsibility it is to rectify the situation, the government or the private sectors? (Ruth and Beauchamp, 1986).

Besides the virtue theory, already described, two other candidates have their defenders. The ethics of caring has been presented as an alternative to traditional bioethics reasoning. Women, it is claimed, embody an ethic of caring, which is itself a prime aim of healing relationships. An ethic of caring would focus on relationships rather than autonomy, on reconciliation rather than winning an argument, and on nurturing rather than imposing dominance (Forester-Miller and Rubinstein, 1992). While the absence of caring relationships is clearly a problem in modern health care, this view has been severely criticized by many, including women, as failing to provide a sufficient basis for replacing ethical principles (Forester-Miller and Rubinstein, 1992).

A final form of analysis is clinical ethics. Its practitioners focus on the clinical realities of moral choices as they emerge in ordinary health care. It is not antithetical to principles but brings abstractions back to reality by measuring proposed solutions against the real world in which doctors and patients live and work. The refusal of treatment on the grounds of futility builds on clinical ethics and real cases. Edmund Pellegrino, a distinguished physician and ethicist, has seen many changes in more than 50 years he has been involved in medicine. Looking toward the future, he does not see the death of principles, but he does foresee some changes. Physicians and other health workers must become familiar with shifts in contemporary moral philosophy if they are to maintain a hand in restructuring the ethics of their profession (Forester-Miller and Rubinstein, 1992).

Medicine and Moral Arguments

Carol Levine narrated this story that in the fall of 1975 a 21-year-old woman lay in a New Jersey hospital-as she had for months in a coma, the victim of a toxic combination of barbiturates and alcohol. Doctors agreed that her brain was irreversibly damaged and that she would never recover. Her parents, after anguished consultation with their priest, asked the doctors and hospital to disconnect the respirator that was artificially maintaining their daughter's life. When the doctors and hospital refused, the parents petitioned the court to make her legal guardian so that they could authorize the withdrawal of treatment. After hearing all the arguments, the court sided with the parents, and the respirator was removed. Contrary to everyone's expectations, however, the young woman did not die but began to breathe on her own, perhaps because, in anticipation of the court order, the nursing staff had gradually weaned her from total dependence on the respirator. She lived for 10 years until her death in June 1985 - comatose, lying in a fetal position, and fed with tubes - in a New Jersey nursing home (Levine, 2008).

The young woman's name was Karen Ann Quinlan, and her case brought national attention to the thorny ethical questions raised by modern medical technology: When, if ever, should life-sustaining technology be withdrawn? Is the sanctity of life an absolute value? What kinds of treatment are really beneficial to a patient in a "chronic vegetative state" like Karen's? And, perhaps the most troubling question, who shall decide? These and similar questions are at the heart of the growing field of biomedical ethics, or as it is usually called *bioethics.*

Carol Levine further stated that ethical dilemmas in medicine are, of course, nothing new. They have been recognized and discussed in Western medicine since a small group of physicians led by Hippocrates on the Isle of Cas in Greece, around the fourth century B.c., subscribed to a code of practice that newly graduated physicians still swear to uphold today. But unlike earlier times, when physicians and scientists had only limited abilities to change the course of disease, today they can intervene in profound ways in the most fundamental processes of life and death. Moreover, ethical dilemmas in medicine are no longer considered the sale province of professionals. Professional codes of ethics, to be sure, offer some guidance, but they are usually unclear and ambiguous about what to do in specific situations. More important, these codes assume that whatever decision is to be made is up to the professional, not the patient. Today, to an ever-greater degree, lay-people patients, families, lawyers, clergy and others want to and have become involved in ethical decision making not only in individual cases, such as the Quinlan case, but also in large societal decisions, such as how to allocate scarce medical resources, including high technology machinery, newborn intensive care units, and the expertise of physicians. While questions about the physician-patient relationship and individual cases are still prominent in bioethics today, the field covers a broad range of other decisions as well, such as the use of reproductive technology, the harvesting and transplantation of organs, equity in access to health care, and the future of animal experimentation (Levine, 2008).

This involvement is part of broader social trends: a general disenchantment with the authority of all professionals and, hence, a greater readiness to challenge the traditional belief that "doctor knows best"; the growth of various civil rights movements among women, the aged, and minorities of which the patients' rights movement is a spin-off; the enormous size and complexity of the health care delivery system, in which patients and families often feel alienated from the professional; the increasing cost of medical care, much of it at public expense; and the growth of the "medical model," in which conditions that used to be considered outside the scope of physicians' control, such as alcoholism and behavioral problems, have come to be considered diseases (Levine, 2008).

Bioethics began in the 1950s as an intellectual movement among a small group of physicians and theologians who started to examine the questions raised by the new medical technologies that were starting to emerge as the result of the heavy expenditure of public funds in medical research after World War II. They were soon joined by a number of philosophers who had become disillusioned with what they saw as the arid abstractions of much analytic philosophy at the time and by lawyers who sought to find principles in the law that would guide ethical decision making or, if such principles were not there, to develop them by case law and legislation or regulation. Although these four disciplines - medicine, theology, philosophy, and law still dominate the field, today bioethics is an interdisciplinary effort, with political scientists, economists, sociologists, anthropologists, nurses, allied health professionals, policymakers, psychologists, and others contributing their special perspectives to the ongoing debates (Forester-Miller and Rubenstein, 1992). The issues that are currently discussed attest to the wide range of bioethical dilemmas, their complexity, and the passion they arouse. But if bioethics today is at the frontiers of scientific knowledge, it is also a field with ancient roots. It goes back to the most basic questions of human life: What is right? What is wrong? How should people act toward others? And why? (Levine, 2008).

Ethics Code

For further understanding of various codes of ethics, I reviewed the Code of Ethics of the American college of Rheumatology which was designed to support the college's mission, and to advance rheumatology through programs of education, research, and advocacy that foster excellence in the care of people with arthritis and rheumatic and musculoskeletal diseases. The Code of Ethics of the American College of Rheumatology applies to the entire College, including its Fellows and Members, and is enforceable solely by the College.

The College can succeed in this mission only if it maintains its reputation in the scientific and medical communities and with the general public as a credible, objective and unbiased force whose statements, activities and relationships are beyond reproach (American Counseling Association, 2005). It is the purpose of this code to provide guidelines that will ensure this reputation is maintained. The College has not attempted in this Code to set forth a position regarding all ethical issues which its members may face in their day-to-day professional activities. The primary purpose of this Code, however, is to emphasize those ethical matters that bear directly on the College's scientific and educational mission and to those activities that relate to that mission.

General Principles of Medical Ethics

These General Principles of Ethics form the first part of this Code of Ethics. These general principles represent generally accepted standards of professional conduct which members should strive to attain. The American College of Rheumatology adopted the following Principles of Professional Conduct and that each member of the College is expected to follow in their relationship with patients, colleagues and the public according to American College of Rheumatology (ACR) (2015, page 2).

1. Members shall be dedicated to providing competent medical care with compassion and respect for human dignity and rights.
2. Members shall uphold the standards of professionalism, be honest in all professional interactions, and strive to report physicians deficient in character or competence, or engaging in fraud or deception, to appropriate entities.
3. Members shall respect the law and also recognize a responsibility to seek changes in those requirements which are contrary to the best interests of the patient.
4. Members shall respect the rights of their patients and shall, within the constraints of the law, safeguard the confidentiality of the physician/patient relationship.
5. Members shall continue to study, apply and advance scientific knowledge, maintain a commitment to medical education and should make useful information available to their patients, colleagues and the public. Physicians have an affirmative obligation to disclose new medical advances to patients and colleagues.

6. Members may choose whom they will serve. In an emergency, however, members should render service to the best of their ability. Having undertaken the care of a patient, a member may not neglect the patient unless the patient has been discharged and may discontinue medical service only after giving adequate notice to the patient.

7. A member's responsibility extends to community and society, and members should participate in civic and community activities contributing to an improved society.

8. Members shall, while caring for a patient, regard responsibility to the patient as paramount.

9. Members shall support access to rheumatologic care for all people.

10. Members shall provide their patients a reasonable explanation of the etiology, treatment and prognosis of their disease.

11. In the practice of medicine, members shall limit the source of their professional income to services actually rendered by them or to the patients under their supervision when they are personally and identifiably responsible for the service. Fees should be commensurate with services rendered, and members shall neither pay nor receive commissions for the referral of patients.

12. Members shall not dispense or supply drugs, remedies or appliances unless it is in the best interest of their patients.

13. Members should seek consultation upon request, in doubtful or difficult cases, or whenever it appears that the quality of medical service may be enhanced thereby.

14. Members should provide the general public information necessary to select a qualified health care provider. Members shall not engage in a false, fraudulent, deceptive or misleading advertising.

15. Members shall ensure that public statements and statements to the press should preserve patient confidentiality and be truthful and not deceptive or misleading.

16. A member's clinical judgment and practice must not be affected by economic interest in, commitment to, or benefit from professionally related commercial enterprises or other actual or potential conflicts of interest. Disclosure of professionally related commercial interests and any other interests that may influence clinical decision-making is required in communications to patients, the public, and colleagues. When a member's interest conflicts

so greatly with the patient's interest as to be incompatible, the member should make alternative arrangements for the care of the patient.

17. In the context of ownership interest in a commercial venture, the member has an obligation to disclose the ownership interest to the patient or referring colleagues prior to utilization; the member's activities must be in strict conformance with the law; and the patient should have free choice to use the member's facility or therapy or to seek the needed services elsewhere (Josen, 1990).

Rules and Policies Pertaining to Volunteers and Staff

1. Members and staff should act in the best interests of the College in carrying out responsibilities in good faith, with reasonable care, honesty, and due diligence.
2. Members and staff shall give individual allegiance to the College when making decisions affecting the College.
3. Members and staff shall not engage in unauthorized activities, i.e. those activities that are not in accordance with College bylaws, policies, and other documents addressing their responsibilities (Josen, 1990).

Policy Regarding Gifts to Members from Industry

Members should be aware that accepting gifts, grants, hospitality or the like may influence clinical judgment. The College recognizes that some gifts given to members by companies in the pharmaceutical, device and medical equipment industries are educationally and socially beneficial. The College also recognizes that certain gifts from industry to physicians and other health professionals, while reflecting customary practices of industry, may not be consistent with accepted principles of medical ethics. In order to avoid the acceptance of inappropriate gifts, the College supports the following Guidelines:

1. Any gifts accepted by members individually should primarily entail a benefit to patients and should not be of substantial value. Accordingly, textbooks, modest meals and other gifts may be

appropriate if they serve a genuine educational function. Cash payments should not be accepted.

2. Individual gifts of minimal value are permissible as long as the gifts are related to the member's work, for example, token items such as pens and notepads.

3. Subsidies to underwrite the costs of continuing medical education conferences or professional meetings can contribute to the improvement of patient care and therefore are permissible. Since the giving of a subsidy directly to a Member by a company's sales representative may create a relationship which could influence the use of the company's products, any subsidy should be accepted by the conference's sponsor who in turn can use the money to reduce the conference's registration fee. Payments to defray the costs of a conference should not be accepted directly from the company by the Members attending the conference.

4. Subsidies from industry should not be accepted to pay for the costs incurred by a member of travel, lodging or other personal expenses of attending conferences or meetings, nor should subsidies be accepted to compensate for the Member's time. Subsidies for hospitality should not be accepted outside of modest meals or social events held as a part of a conference or meeting. It is appropriate for a member who serves as faculty at conferences or meetings to accept reasonable honoraria and to accept reimbursement for reasonable travel, lodging and meal expenses. Token consulting or advisory arrangements cannot be used to justify compensating Members for their time and their travel, lodging and other out-of-pocket expenses.

5. Scholarship or other special funds to permit medical students, residents and fellows to attend carefully selected educational conferences may be permissible as long as the selection of students, residents or fellows who will receive the funds is made by the academic or training institution.

6. No gifts should be accepted if there are strings attached. For example, Members should not accept gifts if they are given in relation to the Members' prescribing practices. In addition, when companies underwrite medical conferences or lectures other than their own, responsibility for and control over the selection of

content, faculty, educational methods and materials should belong to the organizers of the conferences or lectures (Josen, 1990).

American Counseling Association – Ethical Approach

Counselors are often faced with situations that require sound ethical decision-making ability. Determining the appropriate course to take when faced with a difficult ethical dilemma can be a challenge. To assist American Counseling Association (ACA) members in meeting this challenge, the ACA Ethics Committee has developed A Practitioner's Guide to Ethical Decision Making. The intent of this document is to offer professional counselors a framework for sound ethical decision-making. The following will address both guiding principles that are globally valuable in ethical decision making, and a model that professionals can utilize as they address ethical questions in their work.

Moral Principles

Kitchener (1984) has identified five moral principles that are viewed as the cornerstone of our ethical guidelines. Ethical guidelines cannot address all situations that a counselor is forced to confront. Reviewing these ethical principles which are at the foundation of the guidelines often help to clarify the issues involved in a given situation. The five principles, autonomy, non-maleficence, beneficence justice and fidelity are each absolute truths in and of themselves. By exploring the dilemma in regards to these principles, one may come to a better understanding of the conflicting issues.

1. Autonomy is the principle that addresses the concept of independence. The essence of this principle is allowing an individual the freedom of choice and action. It addresses the responsibility of the counselor to encourage clients, when appropriate, to make their own decisions and to act on their own values. There are two important considerations in encouraging clients to be autonomous. First, helping the client to understand how their decisions and their values may or may not be received within the context of the society in which they live, and how they may impinge on the rights of others. The second consideration is related to the client's ability to make sound and rational decisions. People who are not capable of

making competent choices, such as children, and some individuals with mental handicaps should not be allowed to act on decisions that could harm themselves or others.

2. Non-maleficence is the concept of not causing harm to others. Often explained as "above all do no harm", this principle is considered by some to be the most critical of all the principles, even though theoretically they are all of equal weight (Kitchener, 1984; Rosenbaum, 1982; & Stadler, 1986). This principle reflects both the idea of not inflicting intentional harm, and not engaging in actions that risk harming others (Forester-Miller & Rubenstein, 1992).

3. Beneficence reflects the counselor's responsibility to contribute to the welfare of the client. Simply stated it means to do good, to be proactive and also to prevent harm when possible (Forester-Miller & Rubenstein, 1992).

4. Justice does not mean treating all individuals the same. Kitchener (1984) points out that the formal meaning of justice is "treating equals equally and un-equals unequally but in proportion to their relevant differences. If an individual is to be treated differently, the counselor needs to be able to offer a rationale that explains the necessity and appropriateness of treating this individual differently.

5. Fidelity involves the notions of loyalty, faithfulness, and honoring commitments. Clients must be able to trust the counselor and have faith in the therapeutic relationships if growth is to occur. Therefore, the counselor must take care neither to threaten the therapeutic relationship nor to leave obligations unfulfilled.

When exploring an ethical dilemma, one needs to examine the situation and see how each of the above principles may relate to that particular case. At times this alone will clarify the issues enough that the means for resolving the dilemma will become obvious to you. In more complicated cases, it is helpful to be able to work through the steps of an ethical decision making model, and to assess which of these moral principles may be in conflict (Forester & Davis, 1996).

Ethical Decision Making Model

The work of Van Hoose and Paradise (1979), Kitchener (1984), Stadler (1986), Haas and Malouf (1989), Forester-Miller and Rubenstein (1992), and Sileo and Kopala (1993) have been incorporated by Forester & Davis into a practical, sequential, seven steps ethical decision-making model. This model will help alleviate major ethical dilemmas if applied. It was carefully arrived at. A description and discussion of the steps follows (Carol, 2008).

Identify the Problem.

Gather as much information as you can that will illuminate the situation. In doing so, it is important to be as specific and objective as possible. Writing ideas on paper may help you gain clarity. Outline the facts, separating out assumptions, hypotheses, or suspicions. There are several questions you can ask yourself: Is it an ethical, legal, professional, or clinical problem? Is it a combination of more than one of these? If a legal question exists, seek legal advice. Other questions that it may be useful to ask yourself are: Is the issue related to me and what I am or I am not doing? Is it related to a client and/or the client's significant others and what they are or are not doing? Is it related to the institution or agency and their policies and procedures? If the problem can be resolved by implementing a policy of an institution or agency, you can look to the agency's guidelines.

1. It is good to remember that dilemmas you face are often complex, so a useful guideline is to examine the problem from several perspectives and avoid searching for a simplistic solution.
2. Apply the ACA Code of Ethics.
   After you have clarified the problem, refer to the Code of Ethics (ACA, 2005) to see if the issue is addressed there. If there is an applicable standard or several standards and they are specific and clear, following the course of action indicated should lead to a resolution of the problem. To be able to apply the ethical standards, it is essential that you have read them carefully and that you understand their implications. If the problem is more complex and a resolution does not seem apparent, then you probably have

a true ethical dilemma and need to proceed with further steps in the ethical decision making process.

3. Determine the nature and dimensions of the dilemma.
   There are several avenues to follow in order to ensure that on has examined the problem in all its various dimensions.

   o Consider the moral principles of autonomy, non-maleficence, beneficence, justice, and fidelity. Decide which principles apply to the specific situation, and determine which principle takes priority for you in this case. In theory, each principle is of equal value, which means that it is your challenge to determine the priorities when two or more of them are in conflict.

   o Review the relevant professional literature to ensure that you are using the most current professional thinking in reaching a decision.

   o Consult with experienced professional colleagues and/or supervisors. As they review with you the information you have gathered, they may see other issues that are relevant or provide a perspective you have not considered. They may also be able to identify aspects of the dilemma that you are not viewing objectively.

   o Consult your state or national professional associations to see if they can provide help with the dilemma.

4. Generate potential courses of action. Brainstorm as many possible courses of action as possible. Be creative and consider all options. If possible, enlist the assistance of at least one colleague to help you generate options.

5. Consider the potential consequences of all options and determine a course of action. Considering the information you have gathered and the priorities you have set, evaluate each option and assess the potential consequences for all the parties involved. Ponder the implications of each course of action for the client, for others who will be affected, and for yourself as a counselor. Eliminate the options that clearly do not give the desired results or cause even more problematic consequences. Review the remaining options to determine which option or a combination of options best fits the situation and addresses the priorities you have identified.

6. Evaluate the selected course of action. Review the selected course of action to see if it presents any new ethical considerations. Stadler (1986) suggests applying three simple tests to the selected course of action to ensure that it is appropriate. In applying the test of justice, assess your own sense of fairness by determining whether you would treat others the same in this situation. For the test of publicity, ask yourself whether you would want your behavior reported in the press. The test of universality asks you to assess whether you could recommend the same course of action to another counselor in the same situation. If the course of action you have selected seems to present new ethical issues, then one needs to go back to the beginning and reevaluate each step of the process. Perhaps you have chosen the wrong option or you might have identified the problem incorrectly. If one can answer in the affirmative to each of the questions suggested by Stadler, thus passing the tests of justice, publicity, and universality, and satisfied that you have selected an appropriate course of action, then you are ready to move on to implementation.

7. Implement the course of action. Taking the appropriate action in an ethical dilemma is often difficult. The final step involves strengthening your ego to allow you to carry out your plan. After implementing your course of action, it is a good practice to follow up on the situation to assess whether your actions had the anticipated effect and consequences.

It is important to realize that different professionals may implement different courses of action in the same situation. There is rarely one right answer to a complex ethical dilemma. However, if you follow a systematic model, you can be assured that you will be able to give a professional explanation for the course of action you chose. Van Hoose and Paradise (1979) suggest that a counselor is probably acting in an ethically responsible way concerning a client if (1) he or she has maintained personal and professional honesty, coupled with (2) the best interests of the client, (3) without malice or personal gain, and (4) can justify his or her actions as the best judgment of what should be done based upon the current state of the profession (Levine C. 2008).

International Ethical Guidelines

To broaden the understanding of international ethics, I tapped into the International code of ethics for the Occupational Health Professionals in addition to several others. According to Kogi (2002), the aim of occupational health practice is to protect and promote workers' health, to sustain and improve their working capacity and ability to contribute to the establishment and maintenance of a safe and healthy working environment for all, and further promote the adaptation of work to the capabilities of workers, taking into account their state of health. The field of occupational health is broad and covers the prevention of all impairments arising out of employment, work injuries and work-related disorders, including occupational diseases and all aspects relating to the interactions between work and health. In addition, Kogi (2002) mentioned that occupational health professionals should be involved, in the design and choice of health and safety equipment, procedures and safe work practices, and encourage workers' participation in this field and solicit feedback from their experience.

Kogi (2002) also indicated that there are several reasons why the International Commission on Occupational Health (ICOH) has adopted an International Code of Ethics for Occupational Health Professionals, as distinct from codes of ethics for all medical practitioners. One is the increased recognition of the complex and sometimes competing responsibilities of occupational health and safety professionals towards workers, employers, public, public health and labor authorities and other bodies such as social security and judicial authorities. Another reason is the increasing number of occupational health and safety professionals resulting from the compulsory or voluntary establishment of occupational health services. The Code applies to occupational health professionals and occupational health services regardless of whether they operate in a free market context subject to competition or within the framework of public sector health services.

American Public Health Association

According to Thomas, Sage, Dillenberg, and Guillory (2002), the mandate to ensure and protect the health of the public is an inherently moral one. It carries with it an obligation to care for the well being of communities, and it implies the possession of an element of power to carry out that mandate. The need to exercise power to ensure the health of populations while avoiding abuses of such power is at the crux of public health ethics. Until recently, the ethical nature of public health has been implicitly assumed rather than explicitly stated. Increasingly, however, society is demanding explicit attention to ethics (Thomas et al., 2002). This demand arises from technological advances that create new possibilities and, with them, new ethical dilemmas; new challenges to health, such as the advent of HIV; and abuses of power, such as the Tuskegee study of syphilis. Medical institutions have been more explicit about the ethical elements of their practice than public health institutions. However, the concerns of public health are not fully consonant with those of medicine. Thus, we cannot simply translate the principles of medical ethics to public health. In contrast to medicine, public health is concerned more with populations than with individuals, and more with prevention than with cure. The need to articulate a distinct ethic for public health has been noted by a number of public health professionals and ethicists, and that a code of ethics for public health can clarify the distinctive elements of public health and the ethical principles that follow from or respond to those elements (Thomas et al., 2002).

Professional Ethical Conduct for the American Medical Informatics Associations

The American Medical Informatics Association (AMIA) in conjunction with other large professional societies has been working vehemently to promote a strong ethical framework for their membership. The AMIA is a professional home of leading informatics: clinicians, scientists, researchers, educators, students, and other informatics professionals who rely on data to connect people, information, and technology. It is the center of action for more than 5,000 health care professionals, informatics researchers, and thought-leaders in biomedicine, health care, and science. It is an unbiased, authoritative source within the informatics community and the health care industry. AMIA and its members are transforming healthcare through trusted science, education, and practice in biomedical and health informatics (Hurdle et al., 2007). Further, According to Hurdle et. al, (2007), AMIA drives innovation that is defining future approaches to information and knowledge management in biomedical research, clinical care, and public health. As the voice of the nation's top biomedical and health informatics professionals, AMIA members play a leading role in the following:

- moving basic research findings from bench to bedside;
- evaluating interventions across communities;
- assessing the impact of health innovations on health policy; and
- advancing the field of informatics.

Women and minority as research subjects

According to the National Institute of Health (NIH, 2001), it is their policy that women and and members of minority groups and their subpopulations must be included in all NIH-funded clinical research, unless a clear and compelling rationale and justification establishes to the satisfaction of the relevant institute director that inclusion is inappropriate with respect to the health of the subjects or the purpose of the research. Further, cost is not an acceptable reason for exclusion except when the study would duplicate data from other sources.

Investigators, sponsors or ethical review committees should not exclude women of reproductive age from biomedical research. The potential for becoming pregnant during a study should not, in itself, be used as a reason for precluding or limiting participation. However, a thorough discussion of risks to the pregnant woman and to her fetus is a prerequisite for the woman's ability to make a rational decision to enroll in a clinical study. If participation in the research might be hazardous to a fetus or a woman if she becomes pregnant, the sponsors/investigators should guarantee the prospective is subject to a pregnancy test and access to effective contraceptive methods before the research commences. Where such access is not possible, for legal or religious reasons, investigators should not recruit for such possibly hazardous research women who might become pregnant (NIH, 2001). Women in most societies have been discriminated against with regard to their involvement in research. Women who are biologically capable of becoming pregnant have been customarily excluded from formal clinical trials of drugs, vaccines and medical devices owing to concern about undetermined risks to the fetus. Consequently, relatively little is known about the safety and efficacy of most drugs, vaccines or devices for such women, and this lack of knowledge can be dangerous (NIH, 2001).

A general policy of excluding women from such clinical trials is because women are biologically capable of becoming pregnant is unjust in that it deprives women as a class of persons of the benefits of the new knowledge derived from the trials. Further, it is an affront to their right of self-determination. Nevertheless, although women of childbearing age should be given the opportunity to participate in research, they should be helped to understand that the research could include risks to the fetus if they become pregnant during the research. Although this general presumption favors the inclusion of women in research, it must be acknowledged that in some parts of the world women are vulnerable to neglect or harm in research because of their social conditioning to submit to authority, to ask no questions, and to tolerate pain and suffering (NIH, 2001).

Individual consent of women

In research involving women of reproductive age, whether pregnant or non-pregnant, only the informed consent of the woman herself is required for her participation. In no case should the permission of a spouse or partner replace the requirement of individual informed consent (Levin, 2008). If women wish to consult with their husbands or partners or seek voluntarily to obtain their permission before deciding to enroll in research, that is not only ethically permissible but in some contexts highly desirable. A strict requirement of authorization of spouse or partner, however, violates the substantive principle of respect for persons (Levine, 2008).

A thorough discussion of risks to the pregnant woman and to her fetus is a prerequisite for the woman's ability to make a rational decision to enroll in a clinical study (Levine, 2008). For women who are not pregnant at the outset of a study but who might become pregnant while they are still subjects, the consent discussion should include information about the alternative of voluntarily withdrawing from the study and, where legally permissible, terminating the pregnancy (Levine 2008). Further, according to Levine (2008), if the pregnancy is not terminated, they should be guaranteed a medical follow-up. The investigator must establish secure safeguards of the confidentiality of subjects' research data. Subjects should be told the limits, legal or other, to the investigators' ability to safeguard confidentiality and the possible consequences of breaches of confidentiality.

Confidentiality between Investigators and Subjects

According to Parker (2007), research relating to individuals and groups may involve the collection and storage of information that, if disclosed to third parties, could cause harm or distress. Investigators should arrange to protect the confidentiality of such information by, for example, omitting information that might lead to the identification of individual subjects, limiting access to the information, anonymity of data, or other means. During the process of obtaining informed consent the investigator should inform the prospective subjects about the precautions that will be taken to protect confidentiality.

Confidentiality between physician and patient

Patients have the right to expect that their physicians and other health care professional will hold all information about them in strict confidence and disclose it only to those who need or have a legal right to the information, such as other attending physicians, nurses, or other health care workers who perform tasks related to the diagnosis and treatment of patients. A treating physician should not disclose any identifying information about patients to an investigator unless each patient has given consent to such disclosure and unless an ethical review committee has approved such disclosure (Parker, 2007). Physicians and other health care professionals record the details of their observations and interventions in medical and other records. Epidemiological studies often make use of such records. For such studies it is usually impracticable to obtain the informed consent of each identifiable patient; an ethical review committee may waive the requirement for informed consent when this is consistent with the requirements of applicable law and provided that there are secure safeguards of confidentiality (Parker, 2007). In institutions in which records may be used for research purposes without the informed consent of patients, it is advisable to notify patients generally of such practices; notification is usually by means of a statement in patient-information brochures. For research limited to patients' medical records, access must be approved or cleared by an ethical review committee and must be supervised by a person who is fully aware of the confidentiality requirements (Parker, 2007).

Breadth Summary

I broadly presented a review of ethical theories on various issues in health organizations. Theories from John Rawls, Immanuel Kent regarding patients' informed consent and other major ethical dilemmas have been synthesized in this breadth component. Reviewing these ethical frameworks have brought to light the notion that ethical principles are unique to individual organizations although there may be some common grounds for various concepts. In the next two components, however, I strengthen the connection between the aforementioned theoretical frameworks about ethics to specific ethical problems in health care. Further, I provided a review of current research findings regarding ethical implications in health care. This can serve as a reference guide to health care providers.

THE ETHICAL CONSENT

HEALTH SERVICES DELIVERY AND
ETHICAL DECISION-MAKING

In order to acquire a broader and a better understanding of ethical delivery in health services, I reviewed several articles from current research ranging from assessment of harm potential and factors influencing participation decisions to the improvement of patients' health concerns. The ethical concepts reviewed in the breadth components provided a broad understanding of health care ethics. In the depth component, however, a review of current research findings narrowed the focus. The following are the bibliography of contemporary research outcome on ethical issues in health services delivery:

Annotated Bibliography

Blanco and Suresh (2005) found that physicians, nurses, and nurse practitioners underestimated survival rates and overestimated long-term disability rates for intensive premature infants. After education, their estimates of survival and long-term disability rates for these infants improved significantly. They noted that more accurate estimates of survival rates of premature infants by physicians' and nurses' theoretical decision-making appropriateness are required.

A study by Brody and Scherer (2006) on family and physician influence on asthma research participation decisions for adolescents indicated that adolescents were less willing to cede decision making authority to parents than parents anticipated. Parents and adolescents acknowledged a greater openness to influence from physicians than from family for above minimal risk studies, and that Parents were more willing to consider opinions from male adolescents.

To determine the influence of ethical safeguards on research participation, Hammond and Lewis (2004) examined 60 people with schizophrenia, and 69 psychiatrists rated the protectiveness and influence on patients' willingness to participate in research of five safeguards: informed consent, alternative decision makers, institutional review boards, data safety monitoring boards, and confidentiality measures. The investigators found that ethical commitment to research volunteers is expressed in safeguards. These efforts appear to be viewed positively by key stakeholders and may influence research participation decision-making.

Janvier and Barrington (2005) conducted a study to determine the adequacy of records of parental counseling in mothers with threatened preterm delivery before 27 weeks gestation, whether interventions performed at birth were consistent with recorded antenatal decisions, and whether the extent of resuscitation affected the occurrence of serious short-term morbidity. The conclusion was that records of antenatal consultations were often lacking important information. Variations in physician documentation practices are substantial and affect the care offered to infants at the threshold of viability.

To evaluate systematic ethics reflection in groups in community health that includes nursing homes and residencies from the perspectives of employees participating in the groups, the group facilitators, and the service managers, Lillemoen and Pedersen (2015) applied a mixed-methods design with qualitative focus group interviews, observations and written reports at two nursing homes, two home care districts and a residence for people with learning disabilities. The researchers concluded that ethics reflection groups focusing on ethical challenges from the participants' daily work were found to be significant for improved practice, collegial support and cooperation, personal and professional development among staff, facilitators and managers. Further, resources needed to succeed were managerial support, and anchoring ethics sessions in the routine of daily work.

Scherer and Annett (2006) studied the considerable ethical and legal ambiguity surrounding the role of adolescents in the decision-making process for research participation. They examined parent and adolescent perceptions of decision-making authority and sources of influence on adolescent research participation decisions, and examined whether perceptions of influence differed based on adolescent gender and level of research risk. The researchers concluded that adolescents desire responsibility for research participation decisions, though parents may not share these views.

Scott and Kalawish (2004) conducted an electronic and manual literature search for all English-language articles examining the decision-making capacity of elderly persons with dementia or cognitive impairment, reviewing articles in relation to key areas of methodological, clinical, and policy importance. The researchers found that although, incapacity is common, many persons with dementia are capable of making their own medical and research decisions. Furthermore, in early stages of dementia, interventions may improve decisional abilities, and that simple cognitive screenings may be useful by identifying persons in need of more intensive evaluations.

Sharman and Meert (2005) studied the decisions to forgo life support from critically ill children that are commonly faced by parents and physicians, and they identified and described parents' self-reported influences on decisions to forgo life support from their children. The results indicated that previous experience with death and end-of-life decision making for others, their personal observations of their child's suffering, their perceptions of their child's will to survive, their need to protect and advocate for their child, and the family's financial resources and concerns regarding life-long care influence parents decision to forgo life support. The researchers concluded that inclusion of factors like past experiences with end-of-life decisions, and their anticipated emotional adjustments and future resources into discussions is important to parents and may facilitate decisions regarding the limitation or withdrawal of life support.

Clinical Issues in Informed Consent

Appelbaum (2007) stated that law and medical ethics require physicians to obtain the informed consent of their patients before initiating treatment, and that when patients lack the competence to make a decision about treatment, substitute decision makers must be sought. Hence, the determination of whether patients are competent is critical in striking a proper balance between respecting the autonomy of patients who are capable of making informed decisions and protecting those with cognitive impairment. Valid informed consent is premised on the disclosure of appropriate information to a competent patient who is permitted to make a voluntary choice.

Dunn and Roberts (2005) reviewed several publications on the following six topics: professional integrity and sources of potential bias; scientific designs; protocol safeguards; influences on research participation decisions and perceptions of risk; informed consent decision-making capacity, appreciation and the therapeutic misconception, and voluntarism; and informed consent-intervention studies, and found that little empirical work has been conducted on investigator training and potential conflicts of interest. Numerous concepts and controversial issues related to the study designs with the initial focal point being the ethics of placebo-controlled studies have been tackled and that only a handful of reports, however, have empirically addressed these topics, therefore, empirical studies focusing on a variety of ethically relevant domains in schizophrenia research are needed.

In a study to understand mothers' and counselors' perceptions of their roles in decision-making about resuscitation of extremely premature infants at delivery and to assess mothers' and counselors' satisfaction with the counseling and decision-making process, Keenan and Doron (2005) interviewed mothers who delivered an infant between 22 and 27 completed weeks of gestation and their self-identified counselors using a structured interview format. They concluded that decision-making process in this study conforms most closely to a model of informed assent, and that the mothers have been satisfied with this type of counseling because they felt informed and included in the decision-making process. Further, physicians and nurses need to elicit mothers' preferences to incorporate them into the treatment plan, as counseling about the resuscitation of extremely premature infants at delivery is considered directive by mothers even when it is not intended to be directive.

Nijhawan et al. (2013) found that for a drug to get approved and enter into the market it has to prove its safety and efficacy in clinical trials, and that is a research related activities using human being as subjects. Therefore, no one has the right to infract fundamental rights of another person for the sake of fulfilling their own purpose, and that brought about the use of informed consent tool. Informed consent is not only required for clinical trials but an essential prerequisite before enrolling each and every participant in any type of research involving human subjects including; diagnostic, therapeutic, interventional, bioequivalence, social and behavioral studies and for all research conducted domestically or abroad. Obtaining consent involves informing the subject about his or her rights, the purpose of the study, the procedures to be undergone, the potential risks and/or benefits of participation and alternative treatments available if any.

Davis, Berkel and Holcombe (1998) indicated that to ensure that patients fully understand factors related to their care, the Food and Drug Administration (FDA) requires that consent documents contain detailed information regarding eight basic elements of informed consent but little attention has been given to how well patients comprehend these elements, although, health care providers have an ethical and legal responsibility to ensure that patients understand their participation in research. Their study findings raise serious questions regarding the adequacy of the design of written informed consent documents for the substantial proportion of Americans with low-to-marginal literacy skills, and that a high level of reading skill and comprehension is required to understand and complete most consent forms that are required for participation in clinical research studies. The study further indicated that simplifying informed consent material alone makes the forms more appealing and easier to read but will not improve comprehension, and that research is needed to redesign informed consent contents to increase comprehension, especially for participants with inadequate or marginal reading skills.

Annotated Bibliography Summary

It is obvious that ethics in health care delivery yearns for constant monitoring and upgrading as the review indicated. This upgrading involves educating health care providers, patients, and communities to strive for the best in health care delivery. Some of the ethical issues that require immediate attention include the infant survival rate as a result of physicians' estimation influenced by inappropriate record keeping and documentation practices, inadequate intervention services to incapacitated patients so they can make decisions on their own when the need arises, and appropriate parental guidelines to parental decisions to forgo life support of their loved ones at the point of death. Informed consent publications should be free from ambiguity and be more clarity to patients and research subjects.

Further, appropriate ethical protocol should be adhered to in obtaining informed consent from patients prior to initiating treatment.

Literature Review

In addition to the annotated bibliography articles reviewed above, the following articles further provided clarification on the need for further research for a better understanding of ethical decision-making on the part of clinicians and health care providers in general. According to Kim and Karlawish (2002), the importance of research is enormous in that it improves the health of a nation's population as a whole by fostering a better health system. Additionally, emphasis is placed on the devastation of withholding information from patients and research participant. Researchers and health professionals are seriously informed that patients and research participants should be well informed about the risk involve in research participation and or health related procedure.

Global Health and Primary Care Research

A strong primary health care system is essential to provide effective and efficient health care in both resource-rich and resource-poor countries. Although a direct link has not been proven, we can reasonably expect better economic status when the health of the population is improved. Research in primary care is essential to inform practice and to develop better health systems and health policies. Among the challenges for primary care, especially in countries with limited resources, is the need to enhance the research capacity and to engage primary care clinicians in the research enterprise. These caregivers need to be an integral part of the research enterprise so the right questions will be asked - the results from research will be used in practice, and a scholarly and evidence-based approach to primary care will become the norm (Kim & Carlawish, 2002).

The challenge of developing research in primary care can be met only by creating a strong infrastructure. This will include strengthening academic departments, enhancing links to researchers in other fields, improving training programs for future primary care researchers, developing more practice-based primary care research networks, and increasing funding for research in primary care. A greatly increased commitment on the part of international organizations both within and outside of primary care is needed, in particular those organizations involved with funding research. Kim and Carlawish provided suggestions to improve the global primary care research enterprise for the benefit of the world's population.

Withholding Information and Deception

Sometimes, to ensure the validity of research, investigators withhold certain information in the consent process. In biomedical research, this typically takes the form of withholding information about the purpose of specific procedures. For example, subjects in clinical trials are often not told the purpose of tests performed to monitor their compliance with the protocol, since if they knew their compliance was being monitored they might modify their behavior and hence invalidate results. In most such cases, the prospective subjects are asked to consent to remain uninformed of the purpose of some procedures until the research is completed; after the conclusion of the study they are given the omitted information. In other cases, because a request for permission to withhold some information would jeopardize the validity of the research, subjects are not told that some information has been withheld until the research has been completed. Any such procedure must receive the explicit approval of the ethical review committee (Appelbaum, 2007).

According to Van Hoose active deception of subjects is considerably more controversial than simply withholding certain information. Lying to subjects is a tactic not commonly employed in biomedical research. Social and behavioral scientists, however, sometimes deliberately misinform subjects to study their attitudes and behavior. For example, scientists have pretended to be patients to study the behavior of health-care professionals and patients in their natural settings (Van Hoose, 1980).

Some people maintain that active deception is never permissible. Others would permit it in certain circumstances. Deception is not permissible, however, in cases in which the deception itself would disguise the possibility of the subject being exposed to more than minimal risk. When deception is deemed indispensable to the methods of a study the investigators must demonstrate to an ethical review committee that no other research method would suffice; that significant advances could result from the research; and that nothing has been withheld that, if divulged, would cause a reasonable person to refuse to participate (Dunn, Nowrangi, and Jeste, 2006). The ethical review committee should determine the consequences for the subject of being deceived, and whether and how deceived subjects should be informed of the deception upon completion of the research. Such informing, commonly called "debriefing", ordinarily entails explaining the reasons for the deception. A subject who disapproves of having been deceived should be offered an opportunity to refuse to allow the investigator to use information thus obtained. Investigators and ethical review committees should be aware that deceiving research subjects may wrong them as well as harm them; subjects may resent not having been informed when they learn that they have participated in a study under false pretenses. In some studies there may be justification for deceiving persons other than the subjects by either withholding or disguising elements of information. Such tactics are often proposed, for example, for studies of the abuse of spouses or children. An ethical review committee must review and approve all proposals to deceive persons other than the subjects. Subjects are entitled to prompt and honest answers to their questions; the ethical review committee must determine for each study whether others who are to be deceived are similarly entitled (Dunn, Nowrangi, and Jeste, 2006).

Intimidation and Undue Influence

Van Hoose pointed out that intimidation in any form invalidates informed consent. Prospective subjects who are patients often depend for medical care upon the physician/investigator, who consequently has certain credibility in their eyes, and whose influence over them may be considerable, particularly if the study protocol has a therapeutic component. They may fear, for example, that refusal to participate would damage the therapeutic relationship or result in the withholding of health services. The physician/investigator must assure them that their decision on whether to participate will not affect the therapeutic relationship or other benefits to which they are entitled. In this situation the ethical review committee should consider whether a neutral third party should seek informed consent. The prospective subject must not be exposed to undue influence. The borderline between justifiable persuasion and undue influence is imprecise; however, the researcher should give no unjustifiable assurances about the benefits, risks or inconveniences of the research, for example, or induce a close relative or a community leader to influence a prospective subject's decision.

Investigators should be completely objective in discussing the details of the experimental intervention, the pain and discomfort that it may entail, and known risks and possible hazards. In complex research projects it may be neither feasible nor desirable to inform prospective participants fully about every possible risk. They must, however, be informed of all risks that a 'reasonable person' would consider material to making a decision about whether to participate, including risks to a spouse or partner (House, 1980).

Exception to the requirement for informed consent in studies of emergency situations

According to Parker, research protocols are sometimes designed to address conditions occurring suddenly and rendering the patients/subjects incapable of giving informed consent. Examples are head trauma, cardiopulmonary arrest and stroke. The investigation cannot be done with patients who can give informed consent in time and there may not be time to locate a person having the authority to give permission. In such circumstances it is often necessary to proceed with the research interventions very soon after the onset of the condition in order to evaluate an investigational treatment or develop the desired knowledge. As this class of emergency exception can be anticipated, the researcher must secure the review and approval of an ethical review committee before initiating the study. If possible, an attempt should be made to identify a population that is likely to develop the condition to be studied. This can be done readily, for example, if the condition is one that recurs periodically in individuals; examples include grand mal seizures and alcohol binges. In such cases, prospective subjects should be contacted while fully capable of informed consent, and invited to consent to their involvement as research subjects during future periods of incapacitation. If they are patients of an independent physician who is also the physician-researcher, the physician should likewise seek their consent while they are fully capable of informed consent. In all cases in which approved research has begun without prior consent of patients/subjects incapable of giving informed consent because of suddenly occurring conditions, they should be given all relevant information as soon as they are in a state to receive it, and their consent to continued participation should be obtained as soon as is reasonably possible (Parker, 2007).

Before proceeding without prior informed consent, the investigator must make reasonable efforts to locate an individual who has the authority to give permission on behalf of an incapacitated patient. If such a person can be located and refuses to give permission, the patient may not be enrolled as a subject. The researcher and the ethical review committee should agree to a maximum time of involvement of an individual without obtaining either the individual's informed consent or authorization according to the applicable legal system if the person is not able to give consent. If by that time the researcher has not obtained either consent or permission – owing either to a failure to contact a representative or to a refusal of either the patient or the person or body authorized to give permission – the participation of the patient as a subject must be discontinued. The patient or the person or body providing authorization should be offered an opportunity to forbid the use of data derived from participation of the patient as a subject without consent or permission (Parker, 2007).

Justification of children's involvement in biomedical research

The participation of children is indispensable for research into diseases of childhood and conditions to which children are particularly susceptible (cf. vaccine trials), as well as for clinical trials of drugs that are designed for children as well as adults. In the past, many new products were not tested for children though they were directed towards diseases also occurring in childhood; thus children either did not benefit from these new drugs or were exposed to them though little was known about their specific effects or safety in children. Now it is widely agreed that, as a general rule, the sponsor of any new therapeutic, diagnostic or preventive product that is likely to be indicated for use in children is obliged to evaluate its safety and efficacy for children before it is released for general distribution. (Edge and Groves, 1994).

Assent of the child. The willing cooperation of the child should be sought, after the child has been informed to the extent that the child's maturity and intelligence permit. The age at which a child becomes legally competent to give consent differs substantially from one jurisdiction to another; in some countries the "age of consent" established in their different provinces, states or other political subdivisions varies considerably. Often children who have not yet reached the legally established age of consent can understand the implications of informed consent and go through the necessary procedures; they can therefore knowingly agree to serve as research subjects. Such knowing agreement, sometimes referred to as assent, is insufficient to permit participation in research unless it is supplemented by the permission of a parent, a legal guardian or other duly authorized representative (Edge and Groves,1994). Some children, who are too immature to be able to give knowing agreement, or assent, may be able to register a 'deliberate objection', an expression of disapproval or refusal of a proposed procedure. The deliberate objection of an older child, for example, is to be distinguished from the behavior of an infant, who is likely to cry or withdraw in response to almost any stimulus. Older children, who are more capable of giving assent, should be selected before younger children or infants, unless there are valid scientific reasons related to age for involving younger children first.

A deliberate objection by a child to taking part in research should always be respected even if the parents have given permission, unless the child needs treatment that is not available outside the context of research, the investigational intervention shows promise of therapeutic benefit, and there is no acceptable alternative therapy. In such a case, particularly if the child is very young or immature, a parent or guardian may override the child's objections. If the child is older and more nearly capable of independent informed consent, the investigator should seek the specific approval or clearance of the scientific and ethical review committees for initiating or continuing with the investigational treatment. If child subjects become capable of independent informed consent during the research, their informed consent to continued participation should be sought and their decision respected (Edge and Groves,1994).

A child with a likely fatal illness may object or refuse assent to continuation of a burdensome or distressing intervention. In such circumstances parents may press an investigator to persist with an investigational intervention against the child's wishes. The investigator may agree to do so if the intervention shows promise of preserving or prolonging life and there is no acceptable alternative treatment. In such cases, the investigator should seek the specific approval or clearance of the ethical review committee before agreeing to override the wishes of the child (Edge and Groves, 1994).

Permission of a parent or guardian - the investigator must obtain the permission of a parent or guardian in accordance with local laws or established procedures. It may be assumed that children over the age of 12 or 13 years are usually capable of understanding what is necessary to give adequately informed consent, but their consent (assent) should normally be complemented by the permission of a parent or guardian, even when local law does not require such permission. Even when the law requires parental permission, however, the assent of the child must be obtained (Edge and Groves, 1994).

In some jurisdictions, some individuals who are below the general age of consent are regarded as "emancipated" or "mature" minors and are authorized to consent without the agreement or even the awareness of their parents or guardians. They may be married or pregnant or be already parents or living independently. Some studies involve investigation of adolescents' beliefs and behavior regarding sexuality or use of recreational drugs; other research addresses domestic violence or child abuse. For studies on these topics, ethical review committees may waive parental permission if, for example, parental knowledge of the subject matter may place the adolescents at some risk of questioning or even intimidation by their parents. A parent or guardian who gives permission for a child to participate in research should be given the opportunity, to a reasonable extent, to observe the research as it proceeds, so as to be able to withdraw the child if the parent or guardian decides it is in the child's best interests to do so (Edge and Groves, 1994).

Finally Edge and Grove stressed on psychological and medical support. They indicated that research involving children should be conducted in settings in which the child and the parent can obtain adequate medical and psychological support. As an additional protection for children, an investigator may, when possible, obtain the advice of a child's family physician, pediatrician or other health-care provider on matters concerning the child's participation in the research.

Depth Summary

The Depth section integrated ethical concepts of classical theories by John Rawls and Immanuel Kant with the findings of current ethical research. Some of the topics of discussion in the literature review included the research participation decision-making, appropriate delivery of information to participants, and the need for global health and primary care research. Furthermore, some of the current research reviews were on the following topics: Parental involvement in treatment decisions regarding their critically ill child and ethical issues in neonatal intensive care and physicians' practices. The findings of these studies may provide opportunity for physicians to evaluate their practices critically. The application section utilizes the findings of current research in the depth section, especially in the area of ethical implication in clinical practice and research approach and the theoretical concepts reviewed in the breadth component to provide guidelines to health care professionals. Adhering to these guidelines may alleviate some of the ethical dilemmas in health care.

APPLICATION

ETHICAL THEORIES APPLIED IN HEALTH SERVICES

Introduction

To accomplish the objective of recommending an effective approach to ethical dilemma, I considered a further review of additional code of ethics below. I have pointed out in the breadth and depth components the importance of ethical implication in health care and the guidelines to an ethical decision in health care, and health provider's awareness of these guidelines. In the application component, however, I further reviewed ethical models at national and international levels. I reviewed the Australian code of ethics into details to provide an insight on international ethics. Additionally, I culminated with the broad ethical concepts reviewed in the depth component and the current research analyzed in the depth component and provided recommendations and guidelines that could be utilized by the health care industry.

AMA Code of Ethics

Doctors, because of their specialized knowledge and expertise, have a professional responsibility to maintain and improve the health of their patients who, either in a vulnerable state of illness or for the maintenance of their health, entrust themselves to medical care. Over the centuries, doctors have held to a body of ethical principles developed primarily to guide their behavior towards patients, their professional peers and society. The Hippocratic oath was an initial expression of such a code. These codes of ethics as I indicated in the depth component guide doctors to promote the health and well being of their patients and prohibit doctors from behaving, if opportunities arise, in their own self interest. The Australian Medical Association accepts the responsibility for setting the standard of ethical behavior expected of all doctors. The Australian Medical Association Code of Ethics represents the core of fundamental principles that should guide doctors in their professional conduct (AMA 1996). I learned a great deal by reviewing the AMA code of ethics and compare it to health organizations here in the United States. This move has helped in recommending an adequate code of ethics for organizations to adopt. Advancing the scope of medical management brings with it new and challenging ethical problems. The Ethics and Professional Conduct Committee of the Australian Medical Association address these issues and provide revisions of the AMA Code of Ethics from time to time, as appropriate practice that every organization should adopt. Health care professionals under Australian Medical Association have the responsibilities of adhering to the following code of ethics (AMA) (1996).

The Doctor and the Patient – Standard of Care

1. Practice the science and art of medicine to the best of your ability and within the limits of your expertise.
2. Continue self-education to improve your personal standards of medical care.
3. Evaluate your patient completely and thoroughly, maintain accurate contemporaneous clinical records.
4. Ensure that doctors and other health professionals who assist in the care of patients are properly qualified and fully competent to carry out the care.

Respect for Patients

1. Ensure that your professional conduct is above reproach.
2. Do not exploit your patient for sexual, emotional or financial reasons.
3. Treat your patient with compassion and respect for human dignity.

Responsibilities to Patients

1. Do not deny treatment to any patient on the basis of color, race, religion, political beliefs or nature of illness.
2. Respect your patient's right to choose their doctors freely, to accept or reject advice and to make their own educated decisions about treatment or procedures.
3. To enable them to make decisions, educate your patient about the nature of any illness from which they are known to suffer, the probable causes and the available treatments, together with their likely benefits and risks.
4. In general, keep in confidence information derived from your patient, or from a colleague regarding your patient, and divulge it only with the patient's permission, except when a court demands.
5. Recommend only those diagnostic procedures which seem necessary to assist in the care of your patient and only that therapy, which seems necessary for their well being,
6. Recommend to your patient that additional opinions and services be obtained when treatment is not within your expertise.
7. Upon request by your patient, make available to another doctor a report of your findings and treatment.
8. Continue to provide services for an acutely ill patient until your services are no longer required, or until the services of another suitable doctor have been obtained.
9. When a personal moral judgment or religious conscience alone prevents the recommendation of some form of therapy, inform your patient so that they may seek alternative care.
10. Recognize that an established relationship between doctor and patient has a value, which dictates that it should not be disturbed without compelling reasons.
11. Recognize that you may refuse treat a patient only in non-emergency situations, where the patient is given adequate notice of this intention and alternative care is reasonably available. However, the first rule under "Responsibilities to Patients" cannot be overridden.
12. Be responsible in setting an appropriate value on your services, and consider the personal service rendered when determining any fee.

13. Where possible, ensure that your patient is aware of your fees. Be prepared to discuss fees with your patient.
14. Do not refer patients to institutions or services in which you have a financial interest without full disclosure of such interest.

Clinical Research

1. Where possible, accept a responsibility to further medical progress by participating in properly developed clinical research studies involving human subjects.
2. Before participating in such studies, ensure that a responsible independent committee appraises the scientific merit of the clinical research, and that an institutional ethics committee evaluates its ethical implications.
3. Recognize that the well being of subjects always takes precedence over the interests of science or society.
4. Obtain prior consent of all research subjects or their agents, but only after explaining the purpose of the clinical research and any reasonably foreseen health hazards.
5. Advise treating doctors of the involvement of their patients in any research project, the nature of the project and its ethical basis.
6. Recognize that subjects should be allowed to a study at any time.
7. Do not allow a refusal to participate at any stages interfere with the doctor-patient relationship or appropriate treatment and care.
8. Protect the right of doctors to trial, and subject new drug or treatment which may offer reasons for saving life, re-establishing health or alleviating all such cases, fully inform subjects about the drug including the new or unorthodox nature of where applicable.

Clinical Teaching

1. Pass on your professional knowledge and skills to junior colleagues.
2. Before embarking on any clinical teaching involve, explain the nature of the teaching methods of a patient's agreement.
3. Do not allow a refusal to participate in teaching affects the doctor-patient relationship.

4. In any teaching exercise, ensure that the proven diagnostic and therapeutic met your patient's comfort your patient's comfort and dignity are maintained.

The Dying Patient

Always bear in mind the obligation of persevering but, allow death to occur with dignity and comfort, is deemed to be inevitable and where curative appears to be futile.

Transplantation

1. Accept that when brain death has occurred (defined as the irreversible cessation of all functioning of the body including brain stein, unless otherwise defined cellular life in the body may be supported if some parts of the body may be used to prolong life or to improve other people.
2. Recognize the responsibility to provide to the relatives a full disclosure of the intent to transplant organs, the purpose of the procedure and, in the case of the donor, the risks of the procedure.
3. Ensure that the determination of the time of death of any donor patient is made by doctors who are in no way concerned with the transplant procedure or associated with the proposed recipient in a way that may exert any influence upon existence made.

International Instruments and Guidelines

The first international instrument on the ethics of medical research, the Nuremberg Code, was promulgated in 1947 as a consequence of the trial of physicians (The Doctors' Trial) who had conducted atrocious experiments on un-consenting prisoners and detainees during the Second World War. The Code, designed to protect the integrity of the research subject, set out conditions for the ethical conduct of research involving human subjects, emphasizing their voluntary consent to research. The Universal Declaration of Human Rights was adopted by the General Assembly of the United Nations in 1948. To give the Declaration legal as well as moral force, the General Assembly adopted in 1966 the International Covenant on Civil and Political Rights. Article 7 of the Covenant states that "No one shall be subjected to torture or to cruel, inhuman or degrading treatment or punishment. In particular, no one shall be subjected without his free consent to medical or scientific experimentation". It is through this statement that society expresses the fundamental human value that is held to govern all research involving human subjects – the protection of the rights and welfare of all human subjects of scientific experimentation (Kogi, 2002).

Since the publication of the Council for International Organizations of Medical Sciences 1993 Guidelines, several international organizations have issued ethical guidance on clinical trials. This has included, from the World Health Organization, in 1995, Guidelines for Good Clinical Practice for Trials on Pharmaceutical Products; and from the International Conference on Harmonization of Technical Requirements for Registration of Pharmaceuticals for Human Use (ICH), in 1996, Guideline on Good Clinical Practice, designed to ensure that data generated from clinical trials are mutually acceptable to regulatory authorities in the European Union, Japan and the United States of America. The Joint United Nations Program on HIV/AIDS published in 2000 the UNAIDS Guidance Document on Ethical Considerations in HIV Preventive Vaccine Research (Kogi, 2002).

In 2001 the Council of Ministers of the European Union adopted a Directive on clinical trials, which will be binding in law in the countries of the Union from 2004. The Council of Europe, with more than 40 member States, is developing a Protocol on Biomedical Research, which will be an additional protocol to the Council's 1997 Convention on Human Rights and Biomedicine. This is a proof of the vital need of ethical guidelines both at the national and international level (Kogi, 2002).

General Ethical Principles

Health organizations today will benefit a lot by incorporating some of the code of ethics enacted by foreign organizations as I indicated in the Breadth and Death components. All research involving human subjects should be conducted in accordance with three basic ethical principles, namely respect for persons, beneficence and justice. It is generally agreed that these principles, which in the abstract have equal moral force, guide the conscientious preparation of proposals for scientific studies. In varying circumstances they may be expressed differently and given different moral weight, and their application may lead to different decisions or courses of action. The present guidelines are directed at the application of these principles to research involving human subjects (Chima, 2013).

Respect for persons incorporates at least two fundamental ethical considerations, namely: a) Respect for autonomy, which requires that those who are capable of deliberation about their personal choices should be treated with respect for their capacity for self-determination; and b) Protection of persons with impaired or diminished autonomy, which requires that those who are dependent or vulnerable be afforded security against harm or abuse.

Beneficence refers to the ethical obligation to maximize benefits and to minimize harms. This principle gives rise to norms requiring that the risks of research be reasonable in the light of the expected benefits, that the research design be sound, and that the investigators be competent both to conduct the research and to safeguard the welfare of the research subjects. Beneficence further proscribes the deliberate infliction of harm on persons; this aspect of beneficence is sometimes expressed as a separate principle *non-maleficence* (do no harm).

Justice refers to the ethical obligation to treat each person in accordance with what is orally right and proper to give each person what is due to him or her. In the ethics of research involving human subjects, the principal refers primarily to *distributive justice*, which requires the equitable distribution of both the burdens and the benefits of participation in research. Differences in distribution of burdens and benefits are justifiable only if they are based on morally relevant distinctions between persons; one such distinction is vulnerability. "Vulnerability" refers to a substantial incapacity to protect one's own interests owing to such impediments as lack of capability to give informed consent, lack of alternative means of obtaining medical care or other expensive necessities, or being a junior or subordinate member of a hierarchical group. Accordingly, special provision must be made for the protection of the rights and welfare of vulnerable persons (Chima, 2013).

Sponsors of research or investigators cannot, in general, be held accountable for unjust conditions where the research is conducted, but they must refrain from practices that are likely to worsen unjust conditions or contribute to new inequities. Neither should they take advantage of the relative inability of low-resource countries or vulnerable populations to protect their own interests, by conducting research inexpensively and avoiding complex regulatory systems of industrialized countries in order to develop products for the lucrative markets of those countries.

In general, the research project should leave low-resource countries or communities better off than previously or, at least, no worse off. It should be responsive to their health needs and priorities in that any product developed is made reasonably available to them, and as far as possible leave the population in a better position to obtain effective health care and protect its own health. Justice requires also that the research be responsive to the health conditions or needs of vulnerable subjects. The subjects selected should be the least vulnerable necessary to accomplish the purposes of the research. Risk to vulnerable subjects is most easily justified when it arises from interventions or procedures that hold out for them the prospect of direct health-related benefit. Risk that does not hold out such prospect must be justified by the anticipated benefit to the population of which the individual research subject is representative (Wirshing and Liberman, 1998).

Informed Consent's General Considerations

Informed consent is a decision to participate in research, taken by a competent individual who has received the necessary information; who has adequately understood the information; and who, after considering the information, has arrived at a decision without having been subjected to coercion, undue influence or inducement, or intimidation. Informed consent is based on the principle that competent individuals are entitled to choose freely whether to participate in research. Informed consent protects the individual's freedom of choice and respects the individual's autonomy. As an additional safeguard, it must always be complemented by independent ethical review of research proposals. This safeguard of independent review is particularly important as many individuals are limited in their capacity to give adequate informed consent; they include young children, adults with severe mental or behavioral disorders, and persons who are unfamiliar with medical concepts and technology (Wirshing and Liberman, 1998).

It is advisable for Health care providers to be familiar with the following guidelines when making ethical decisions as recommended by committee members: **Process** - Obtaining informed consent is a process that is begun when initial contact is made with a prospective subject and continues throughout the course of the study. By informing the prospective subjects, by repetition and explanation, by answering their questions as they arise, and by ensuring that each individual understands each procedure, investigators elicit their informed consent and in so doing manifest respect for their dignity and autonomy. Each individual must be given as much time as is needed to reach a decision, including time for consultation with family members or others. Adequate time and resources should be set aside for informed-consent procedures (Appelbaum, 2007).

Language - Informing the individual subject must not be simply a ritual recitation of the contents of a written document. Rather, the investigator must convey the information, whether orally or in writing, in language that suits the individual's level of understanding. The investigator must bear in mind that the prospective subject's ability to understand the information necessary to give informed consent depends on that individual's maturity, intelligence, education and belief system. It depends also on the investigator's ability and willingness to communicate with patience and sensitivity.

Comprehension - The investigator must then ensure that the prospective subject has adequately understood the information. The investigator should give each one full opportunity to ask questions and should answer them honestly, promptly and completely. In some instances the investigator may administer an oral or a written test or otherwise determine whether the information has been adequately understood.

Documentation of consent - Consent may be indicated in a number of ways. The subject may imply consent by voluntary actions, express consent orally, or sign a consent form. As a general rule, the subject should sign a consent form, or, in the case of incompetence, a legal guardian or other duly authorized representative should do so. The ethical review committee may approve waiver of the requirement of a signed consent form if the research carries no more than minimal risk – that is, risk that is no more likely and not greater than that attached to routine medical or psychological examination – and if the procedures to be used are only those for which signed consent forms are not customarily required outside the research context. Such waivers may also be approved when existence of a signed consent form would be an unjustified threat to the subject's confidentiality. In some cases, particularly when the information is complicated, it is advisable to give subjects information sheets to retain; these may resemble consent forms in all respects except that subjects are not required to sign them. The ethical review committee should clear their wording. When consent has been obtained orally, investigators are responsible for providing documentation or proof of consent (Appelbaum, 2007).

Waiver of the consent requirement - Investigators should never initiate research involving human subjects without obtaining each subject's informed consent, unless they have received explicit approval to do so from an ethical review committee. However, when the research design involves no more than minimal risk and a requirement of individual informed consent would make the conduct of the research impracticable (for example, where the research involves only excerpting data from subjects' records), the ethical review committee may waive some or all of the elements of informed consent.

Renewing consent - When material changes occur in the conditions or the procedures of a study, and also periodically in long-term studies, the investigator should once again seek informed consent from the subjects. For example, new information may have come to light, either from the study or from other sources, about the risks or benefits of products being tested or about alternatives to them. Subjects should be given such information promptly. In many clinical trials, results are not disclosed to subjects and investigators until the study is concluded. This is ethically acceptable if an ethical review committee has approved their non-disclosure.

Cultural considerations - In some cultures an investigator may enter a community to conduct research or approach prospective subjects for their individual consent only after obtaining permission from a community leader, a council of elders, or another designated authority. Such customs must be respected. In no case, however, may the permission of a community leader or other authority substitute for individual informed consent. In some populations the use of a number of local languages may complicate the communication of information to potential subjects and the ability of an investigator to ensure that they truly understand it. Many people in all cultures are unfamiliar with, or do not readily understand, scientific concepts such as those of placebo or randomization. Sponsors and investigators should develop culturally appropriate ways to communicate information that is necessary for adherence to the standard required in the informed consent process. Also, they should describe and justify in the research protocol the procedure they plan to use in communicating information to subjects. For collaborative research in developing countries, the research project should, if necessary, include the provision of resources to ensure that informed consent can indeed be obtained legitimately within different linguistic and cultural settings (Appelbaum, 2007).

Use of medical records and biological specimens - Medical records and biological specimens taken in the course of clinical care may be used for research without the consent of the patients/subjects only if an ethical review committee has determined that the research poses minimal risk, that the rights or interests of the patients will not be violated, that their privacy and confidentiality or anonymity are assured, and that the research is designed to answer an important question and would be impracticable if the requirement for informed consent were to be imposed. Patients have a right to know that their records or specimens may be used for research. Refusal or reluctance of individuals to agree to participate would not be evidence of impracticability sufficient to warrant waiving informed consent. Records and specimens of individuals who have specifically rejected such uses in the past may be used only in the case of public health emergencies (Appelbaum, 2007)**.**

Recommended Guidelines for Obtaining Informed Consent

According to Rao (2008), before requesting an individual's consent to participate in research, the investigator must provide the following information, in language or another form of communication that the individual can understand: These guidelines will alleviate problems that arise in ethical decision making by professional inpatients selection or participants for a research study.

1. that the individual is invited to participate in research, the reasons for considering the individual suitable for the research, and that participation is voluntary;
2. that the individual is free to refuse to participate and will be free to withdraw from the research at any time without penalty or loss of benefits to which he or she would otherwise be entitled;
3. the purpose of the research, the procedures to be carried out by the investigator and the subject, and an explanation of how the research differs from routine medical care;
4. for controlled trials, an explanation of features of the research design (e.g., randomization, double-blinding), and that the subject will not be told of the assigned treatment until the study has been completed and the blind has been broken;

5. the expected duration of the individual's participation (including number and duration of visits to the research center and the total time involved) and the possibility of early termination of the trial or of the individual's participation in it;

6. whether money or other forms of material goods will be provided in return for the individual's participation and, if so, the kind and amount;

7. that, after the completion of the study, subjects will be informed of the findings of the research in general, and individual subjects will be informed of any finding that relates to their particular health status;

8. that subjects have the right of access to their data on demand, even if these data lack immediate clinical utility (unless the ethical review committee has approved temporary or permanent non-disclosure of data, in which case the subject should be informed of, and given, the reasons for such non-disclosure);

9. any foreseeable risks, pain or discomfort, or inconvenience to the individual (or others) associated with participation in the research, including risks to the health or well-being of a subject's spouse or partner;

10. the direct benefits, if any, expected to result to subjects from participating in the research;

11. the expected benefits of the research to the community or to society at large, or contributions to scientific knowledge;

12. whether, when and how any products or interventions proven by the research to be safe and effective will be made available to subjects after they have completed their participation in the research, and whether they will be expected to pay for them;

13. any currently available alternative interventions or courses of treatment;

14. the provisions that will be made to ensure respect for the privacy of subjects and for the confidentiality of records in which subjects are identified;

15. the limits, legal or other, to the investigators' ability to safeguard confidentiality, and the possible consequences of breaches of confidentiality;

16. policy with regard to the use of results of genetic tests and familial genetic information, and the precautions in place to

prevent disclosure of the results of a subject's genetic tests to immediate family relatives or to others (e.g., insurance companies or employers) without the consent of the subject;

17. the sponsors of the research, the institutional affiliation of the investigators, and the nature and sources of funding for the research;

18. the possible research uses, direct or secondary, of the subject's medical records and of biological specimens taken in the course of clinical care;

19. whether it is planned that biological specimens collected in the research will be destroyed at its conclusion, and, if not, details about their storage (where, how, for how long, and final disposition) and possible future use, and that subjects have the right to decide about such future use, to refuse storage, and to have the material destroyed;

20. whether commercial products may be developed from biological specimens, and whether the participant will receive monetary or other benefits from the development of such products;

21. whether the investigator is serving only as an investigator or as both investigator and the subject's physician;

22. the extent of the investigator's responsibility to provide medical services to the participant;

23. that treatment will be provided free of charge for specified types of research-related injury or for complications associated with the research, the nature and duration of such care, the name of the organization or individual that will provide the treatment, and whether there is any uncertainty regarding funding of such treatment.

24. In what way, and by what organization, the subject or the subject's family or dependents will be compensated for disability or death resulting from such injury or, when indicated, that there are no plans to provide such compensation;

25. whether or not, in the country in which the prospective subject is invited to participate in research, the right to compensation is legally guaranteed;

26. That an ethical review committee has approved or cleared the research protocol.

Discussions

Ethics is the moral principle act of conducting oneself appropriately (Forester-Miller and Rueinstein, 1992). I have presented ethical approaches by several institutions such as, healthcare, colleges, and international agencies. The codes of ethics guiding institutions are unique but the bottom line of each one of them is to reduce if not eliminate harm to mankind. We have seen how the National Commission for the Protection of Human Subjects of Biomedical and Behavioral Research grappled with some of the most difficult issues facing researchers and society: When, if ever, is it ethical to do research on children, or on people with mental problems? Furthermore, at international level, I referred to the Belmont Report of 1978, where the commissioners' outline emphasized on the respect for persons, beneficence, and justice as the three items that should govern the conduct of research with human beings (Belmont Report, 1978). These three principles, they believed, are generally accepted in our cultural tradition and can serve as basic justifications for the many particular ethical prescriptions and evaluations of human action (Belmont Report, 1978).

One of the strains of ethical theory that is prominent in bioethics is natural law theory, first developed by St. Thomas Aquinas (1223-1274). According to this theory, actions are morally right if they accord with our nature as human beings. The attribute that is distinctively human is the ability to reason and to exercise intelligence (Berg and Bradddock, 2001). Thus, argues this theory, we can know the good, which is objective and can be learned through reason. References to natural law theory are prominent in the works of Catholic theologians and writers as I pointed out earlier. They see natural law as ultimately derived from God but knowable through the efforts of human beings. The influence of natural law theory can be seen in various health issues such as the one on human stem cell research.

The issue of confidentiality is another area that warrants attention in health and other institutions. According to Parker (2007), research relating to individuals and groups may involve the collection and storage of information that, if disclosed to third parties, could cause harm or distress. Investigators are advised to protect the confidentiality of patients at all cost. During the process of obtaining informed consent the investigator should inform the prospective subjects in research about the precautions that will be taken to protect confidentiality. Additionally, patients have the right to expect that their physicians and other health care professionals will hold all information about them in strict confidence and disclose it only to those who need, and or have a legal right to the information. A treating physicians and their assistance should not disclose any identifying information about patients to an investigator unless each patient has given consent to such disclosure and unless an ethical review committee has approved such disclosure.

REFERENCES

ABA Commission on law and aging. (2007). Surrogate consent in the absence of an advance directive. Chicago: *American Bar Association.*

American College of Rheumatology (ARC, 2015). Education – Treatment – Research. Retrieved from http://www.rheumatology.org/about_us

American counseling association (2005). Code of ethics. *Alexandra*, VA.

Appelbaum P. (2007). Assessment of patients' competence to consent to treatment. *The New England Journal of Medicine.* Vol. 357:1634-1640.

Australian Medical Association (AMA) (1996). *Code of Ethics.*

Blanco F. and Suresh G. (2005). Ensuring accurate knowledge of prematurity outcomes for prenatal counseling. *Division of Neonatology, Department of Pediatrics*, Vermont Children's Hospital, University of Vermont, Burlington, Vermont, USA.

Barry M. (2000). Involving patients in medical decisions: How can physicians do better? *Journal of American Medical Association.*

Bayles M. (1981). Professional ethics. Belmont, CA: *Wada worth Publishing.*

Belmont Report (1978). *National commission for the protection of human rights*

Berg A. and Braddock C. (2001). Informed consent: *Legal theory and clinical practice.* New York: Oxford University Press.

Brody J. and Scherer D. (2006). Family and physician influence on asthma research participation decisions for adolescents: the effects of adolescent gender and research risk. *Center for Family and Adolescent Research, Oregon Research Institute.*

Bruhn J. & Handerson G. (1991). Values in health care: *Choices and conflicts.* Springfield IL: Charles C. Thomas, Publisher.

Carpenter W. and Lahti A. (2000). Decisional capacity for informed consent in Schizophrenia Research. *General Psychiatry* 57:533-538.

Chima S. (2013). Evaluating the quality of informed consent and contemporary clinical practices by medical doctors in South Africa: *An empirical study. BMC Medical Ethics,* 14(1). Doi: 10.1186/1472-6939-14-S1-S3.

Darr K. (1997). Ethics in health service management. 3rd Ed. Baltimore, MD: *Health Profession Press.*

Davis T., Berkel H., and Holcombe R. (1998). Informed Consent for Clinical Trials: *a Comparative Study of Standard Versus Simplified Forms.* Oxford Journal of Medicine and Health, National Cancer Institute. Vol. 90, issue 9. 668-674. Doi: 10.1093/jnci/90.9668.

Dixon J. and Smalley M. (1981). *The Surgical/ethical challenge.* 246(27): 2471-2.

Dunn B. and Roberts W. (2005). Emerging findings in ethics of schizophrenia research. *Department of Psychiatry,* University of California at San Diego, USA.

Dunn L., Nowrangi M., and Jeste D. (2006). Assessing decisional capacity for clinical research or treatment: A Review of Instruments. *AM J Psychiatry,* 163: 1323 -1334.

Edge S. & Groves R. (1994). The Ethics of Health Care: A guide to clinical practice. Albany, NY: Delmar Publishers, Inc. Etchells E. and Katz M. (1997). Accuracy of clinical impressions and mini-mental state exam scores for assessing capacity to consent to major medical treatment. *Psychosomatics;* 38:239-245.

Farnsworth M. (1990). Competency evaluations in a general hospital. *Psychosomatics* Vlo. 31: 70-76.

Fitten J. and Hamman C. (1990). Assessing treatment decision-making capacity in elderly nursing home residents. *Geriatric Soc*: 38, 1097-1104.

Fisher S. and Alexandra D. (1983). The social organization of doctor-patient communication. Washington DC: *Center for Applied Linguistics.*

Forester H. and Davis T. (1996). A practitioner's guide to ethical decision making. *American Counseling Association.*

Forester-Miller H and Rubenstein L. (1992). Group counseling: *Ethics and professional Issues.* Denver, CO: Love Publishing Co.

Goodwin P. and Lair T. (1995). Decision-making incapacity among nursing home residents. NMS Survey. *Behavior Science Law,* 13:405-414.

Haas J. and Malouf L. (1989). Keeping up the good work: A practitioner's guide to mental health ethics. Sarasota FL: *Professional Resource Exchange, Inc.*

Hammond K. and Lewis R. (2004). Influence of ethical safeguards on research participation: comparison of perspectives of people with schizophrenia and psychiatrists. *Department of Psychiatry and Behavioral Medicine.*

Hurdle J, et al., (2007). A Code of Professional Ethical Conduct for the American Medical Informatics Association. *J Am Med Inform Assoc.* 14(4): 391–393. Doi: 10.1197/jamia.M2456.

Janvier A. and Barrington K. (2005). The ethics of neonatal resuscitation at the margins of viability: informed consent and outcomes. *Division of Neonatology, Royal Victoria Hospital*, Montreal, Quebec, Canada.

Josen A. (1990). The new medicine and the old ethics. Cambridge, MA: Harvard University Press.

Katz J. (1984). The silent world of doctor and patient. *New York: Free Press.*

Keenan H. and Doron M. (2005). Comparison of mothers' and counselors' perceptions of pre-delivery counseling for extremely premature infants. *Department of Social Medicine,* University of North Carolina.

Kichener K. (1984). Intuition, critical evaluation and ethical principles: *The foundation for ethical decisions in counseling psychology.* Counseling Psychologist, 12(3), 43-55.

Kim H. and Swan J. (2007). Determining when impairment constitutes incapacity for informed consent in schizophrenia research. *Br J Psychiatry*; 191:38-43.

Kim S. and Karlawish J. (2002). Current state of research on decision-making competence of cognitively impaired elderly persons. *Geriatric Psychiatry* 10:151-165.

Kitchener S. (1984). Intuition critical evaluation and ethical principles: *The Foundation for Ethical Decision in Counseling Psychology.* Counseling Psychologist, 12(3), 43-55.

Kogi K, (2002). International Code of Ethics for Occupational Health Professionals (ICOH). Retrieved from http://wwwicohweb.org/core_ethics_eng.pdf.

Levine C. (2008). Taking sides. *Clashing view on bioethicaliIssues.* McGraw-Hill Companies, Inc.

Lillemoen L and Pedersen R (2015). Ethics reflection groups in community health services: an evaluation study. University of Oslo. *BMC Medical Ethics.* Doi:10.1186/s12910-015-0017-9.

McKinnon K. Cournos F. (1989). Rivers in practice: clinicians' assessments of patients' decision-making capacity. *Hosp Community Psychiatry*; 40:1159-1162.

National Institute of Health (NIH, 2001). NIH policy and guidelines on the inclusion of women and minorities as subjects in clinical research. US Department Health and Human Services. Retrieved from grants.nih. gov/grants/fundingwomen_min/guidelines_amended_10_2001 htm

Nijhawan L et al. (2013). Informed consent: Issues and challenges. Journal of Adv Pharm Technol Res. 4(3): 134–140. Doi: 10.4103/2231-4040.116779

Parker L. (2007). Informed Consent: *Legal theory and clinical practice.* New York: Oxford University Press.

Rao S. (2008). Informed consent: *An ethical obligation or legal compulsion?* Journal of Cutaneous and Aesthetic Surgery. 1(1): 33-35. Doi: 10.4103/0974-41159.

Rawls J. (1971). A theory of justice. Cambridge MA: *The Belknap Press.*

Rogerson K. (1991). Introduction to ethical theory. Fort Worth, TX: *Holt, Rinehard and Winston, Inc.*

Rosenbaum M. (1982). Ethical problems of group psychotherapy. *Ethics and values Guidebook*: New York Free Press.

Ruth R. and Beauchamp T. (1986). A History and theory of informed consent. New York: *Oxford University Press.* Saks E., Dunn L., Marshall B. (2002). A new instrument to measure the appreciation component of capacity to consent to research. *Am J Geriatric Psychiatry* 2002; 10:166-174.

Scherer D. and Annett R. (2006)). Family and physician influence on asthma research participation decisions for adolescents: the effects of adolescent gender and research risk. Center for Family and Adolescent Research, *Oregon Research Institute.*

Scott Y. and Kalawish M. (2004). Current State of Research on Decision-Making Competence of Cognitively Impaired Elderly Persons. *American Association for Geriatric Psychiatry.*

Sharman M. and Meert K. (2005). What influences parents' decisions to limit or withdraw life support. Department of Pediatrics, Children's Hospital ofMichigan, *Wayne State University, Detroit.*

Sileo F. & Kopala M. (1993). An A-B-C-D-E Worksheet for promoting beneficence when considering ethical issues. *Counseling and Values*, 37, 89-95.

Singer P. (1994). Rethinking life and death. *The collapse of our traditional Ethics*. New York: St. Martin's Press.

SophiaOmni (2012). Sophia Project. On the supposed right to lie from benevolent motives. *Immanuel Kant*. Retrieved from www. sophiaoomni.org

Stadler H. (1986). Making Hard Choices: Clarifying Controversial ethical issues. *Counseling and Human Development*, 19, 1-10.

The council for international organizations of medical sciences (CIOMS). (2002). *International ethical guidelines for biomedical research involving human subjects.*

Thomas, C., Sage M., Dillenberg J. and Guillory J. (2002). A Code of Ethics for Public Health. *American Public Health Association (APHA)*. Am J Public Health. 92(7): 1057-1059.

Van Hoose W. (1980). Ethics and counseling. *And human development*, 13(1), 1-12.

Vollmann J. and Danker H (2003). Competence of mentally ill patients: *a comparative empirical study*. Psychol Med; 33:1463-1471

Wirshing DA, Wirshing WC, Marder SC, Liberman RP, Mintz J. Informed consent: assessment of comprehension. *Am J Psychiatry* 1998; 155:1508-1511.

www.ingramcontent.com/pod-product-compliance
Lightning Source LLC
Chambersburg PA
CBHW021020180526
45163CB00005B/2049